Healthy Heart

GW00716587

CONTENTS

(072-12571)

© Ian Banks 2012

Revision date: March 2015

Cartoons by Jim Campbell

Cover photograph
© iStockphoto.com/Franz-W Franzelin

ISBN: 978 0 85761 034 8

The Information Standard	This organisation has been certified as a producer of reliable health and social care information.
Certified member	www.theinformationstandard.org

The MHF encourage your comments and feedback:
http://www.malehealth.co.uk/MMfeedback

A full list of the references used in this mini manual is available at:
http://www.malehealth.co.uk/MMreferences

Printed in the UK.

Haynes Publishing, Sparkford, Yeovil, Somerset BA22 7JJ, England

Haynes North America, Inc, 861 Lawrence Drive, Newbury Park, California 91320, USA

Haynes Publishing Nordiska AB, Box 1504, 751 45 Uppsala, Sweden

The author and the publisher have taken care to make sure that the advice given in this edition is right at the time of publication. We advise you to read and understand the instructions and information included with all medicines we recommend, and to carefully consider whether a treatment is worth taking. The author and the publisher have no legal responsibility for the results of treatments, misuse or over-use of the remedies in this book or their level of success in individual cases.

The author and the publisher do not intend this book to be used instead of advice from a medical practitioner, which you should always get for any symptom or illness.

Introduction

Being a heart is a man-sized job these days. Hearts tend to get forgotten, even taken for granted. Bad idea. Clench your fist. Stick it in the middle of your chest. Yep, that's about the length and breadth of a lump of muscle which can never rest, designed only for action. There's absolutely nothing it likes better than a challenge, getting its valves ticking and blood rushing to every part of the body.

- But only at the right pressure and with time to slow down
- On the correct, poison-free fuel
- With no sticky lumps to block it up.

It's a top of the range, high performance pump but it ain't maintenance-free. Give it what it wants and it'll last you a long life time without replacement.

This is your Heart Manual for man pumps. Keep it in your glove box of life, show it to your mates, use it to wipe your dip stick but most of all, read it. Cover to cover. It might just save you breaking your heart.

During an average life time, the heart will pump 55 million gallons of blood. That's:
- A quarter of a billion litres
- The amount of oil carried by the Exxon Valdez when it sank off Alaska in 1989
- 1 million domestic baths or 100 Olympic-sized swimming pools.

Hearty food

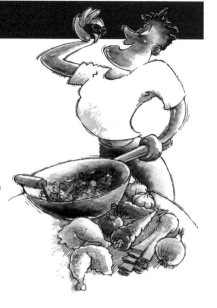

Eating a well-balanced diet can improve your health by:

• Keeping your weight down
• Lowering your blood cholesterol
• Preventing high blood pressure.

All of these lower your risk of getting heart disease and help prevent things like diabetes and cancer.

See www.malehealth.co.uk/diet

Fat facts

You do need to eat a little fat because it helps the body soak up some vitamins, boosts energy and supplies some of the things the body can't make itself, such as vitamins and building blocks for hormones. But too much fat means too much weight.

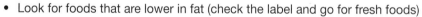

• Look for foods that are lower in fat (check the label and go for fresh foods)
• Fish and chips won't kill you, but eating high fat foods all the time can seriously damage your health
• Cut down on the fat you use in cooking. Grill, casserole or stew meat instead of frying it.

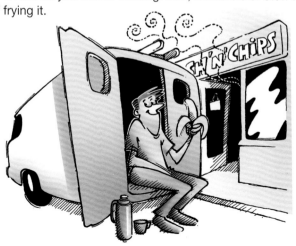

Boring? I'll eat my hat

Eating well doesn't need to be boring. Eating a good variety of food makes sense and can be very tasty too. Basically you need:

- More fruit and vegetables
- Some starchy foods such as rice, bread, pasta and potatoes
- Less saturated fat, salt and sugar
- Some protein-rich foods such as fresh meat, fish, eggs and pulses.

Salt and increased blood pressure

Eating too much salt can raise your blood pressure. People with high blood pressure are three times more likely to develop heart disease or have a stroke than people with normal blood pressure.

Tips to reduce salt

- Eat home-cooked meals rather than ready meals when possible
- Use fresh fish and lean meat, rather than canned, smoked or processed meat, helping to reduce fat as well
- Go for food with low or reduced sodium levels or no added salt
- Cook rice, pasta and hot cereals without salt
- Use herbs and spices instead of salt when cooking.

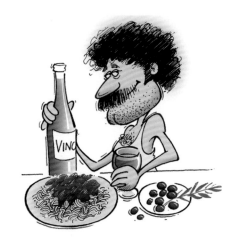

Fruit and veg

Unless you have been hiding under a rock for the past few years you will know that eating plenty of fruit and vegetables is good for your health. Aim to eat at least five portions a day.

Heavyweight issues

Did you know that:

- Men with waist sizes over 40 inches are 33% more likely to die from cancer than those who are a healthy weight
- 2 out of every 5 people in the United Kingdom have high blood pressure which is often linked to being overweight
- A person who is 12 kg (about two stone) overweight is twice as likely to have a heart attack as someone who is a healthy weight
- Every year, 30,000 deaths are directly linked to obesity, and every 17 1/2 minutes a person dies of an obesity-related illness.

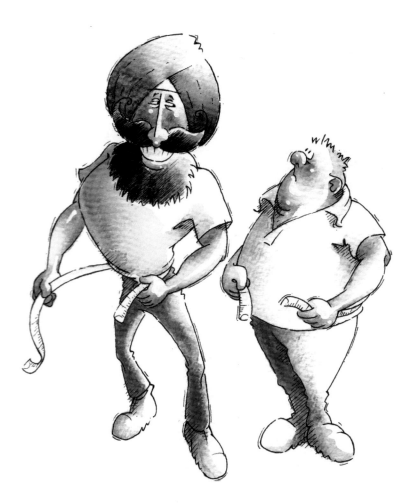

Good gut size

Men with a waist size of more than 94 centimetres (37 inches) have increased health risks. A waist measurement of over 102 centimetres (40 inches) can lead to serious health risks.

African-Caribbean and Asian men have an increased risk of developing diabetes, high blood pressure and heart disease, and being overweight increases this risk. Being 40 years old is fine, having a 40-inch waist isn't.

How to measure your waist

- Find the top of your hip bone and the bottom of your ribs
- Breathe out naturally
- Place the tape measure between these points and wrap it around your waist
- Make a note of the measurement.

Coronary heart disease (CHD)

Coronary crowns

- Hold out your hand as if to pick up a grapefruit
- Your fingers are the ring or 'crown' of arteries, blood vessels, surrounding the heart supplying oxygen and sugar to drive the muscle
- Blocked coronary arteries (CHD) are the most common cause of male early death in Europe
- CHD is preventable and declining as people increasingly give up smoking.

1   Coronary arteries
2   Blockage
3   Oxygen-starved tissue

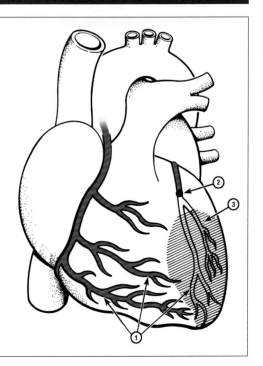

Chest pain (angina)

Fat builds up inside the artery wall, reducing its flexibility and roughing up the smooth inner surface. The artery gradually gets narrower, cutting down the amount of fuel available for the heart muscle. Not surprisingly this causes pain (angina) during exercise when the muscle needs more blood.

Heart attack (myocardial infarction, MI)

Small mounds of fat build up on the artery walls. If one of these mounds breaks off it will tumble through your artery until it becomes blocked in a narrower or already partially-blocked part of the artery. The result can be fatal. Starved of oxygen the heart muscle will die unless the block is removed quickly. In men, this usually hurts, pain moves up from the chest into the neck or left shoulder. But beware, sometimes there is little pain, just a vague feeling of sickness and shortness of breath. If there is severe damage, the heart can actually stop beating. Quick action can keep blood flowing to the brain and lungs (see page 16 *Hard & Fast*) until medical help arrives.

Chip off the old block

Only men have the Y chromosome which might be bad luck when it comes to heart attacks. A recent British Heart Foundation study shows men who inherit certain genes, found only on the Y male chromosome, are more likely to suffer from heart disease.

- This helps explain why these conditions tend to run in families but only in men
- The race is now on to develop screening tests to identify which men are at increased risk.

So it's important for *all* men to get their risks down.

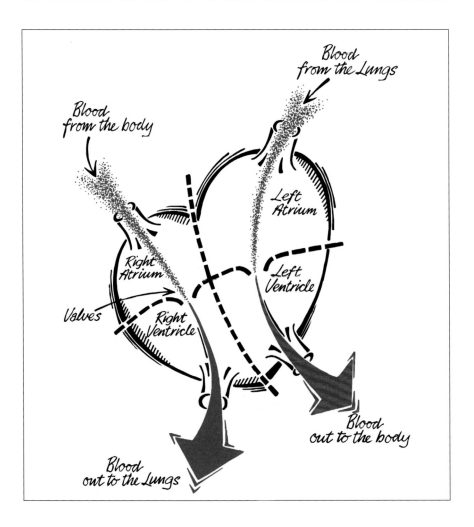

Blood from the Lungs

Blood from the body

Left Atrium

Right Atrium

Left Ventricle

Valves

Right Ventricle

Blood out to the body

Blood out to the Lungs

High blood pressure (hypertension)

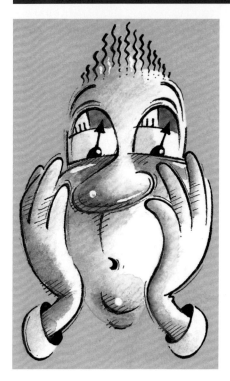

High blood pressure (hypertension) is rightly called the 'Silent Killer' because there are very few signs that things are going wrong. A car tyre can look perfectly fine yet may be at a dangerous pressure. You only know if you actually check the pressure. The same applies to your blood pressure. A tyre at the wrong pressure can blow out on the motorway or hard cornering at speed.

Blood pressure varies throughout the day. This is normal, and whether you have high blood pressure or not. Blood pressure responds to activity or rest. As you get older blood pressure tends to rise. High blood pressure is more common among people of African-Caribbean descent. Diabetes and other illnesses are also associated with raised blood pressure.

Hearts are not 'rotary pumps' like you find in washing machines or the oil pump in a car engine. With each beat hearts have to pump a load of blood out to the body then fill up ready for the next beat. Blood pressure is about both of these things and is given as two numbers. One for when the heart is pumping and the other while it is being refilled. So the first pressure is always higher than the first and you will see numbers like 120/80.

Why is high blood pressure dangerous?

Having too high a blood pressure for too long can cause a stroke or heart attack.

High blood pressure for too long also puts a strain on blood vessels all over the body, especially those going to the brain. It can damage the lining of arteries which can then block up or burst causing a stroke.

High blood pressure is a frequent cause and complication of kidney disease. This affects over 1 in 10 men (HSE 2010) and can easily be detected by a simple blood and urine protein test.

Routine maintenance

After seeing your pharmacist or practice nurse, buy a simple blood pressure monitor. They can be bought for as little as £10 and are very good, but you should also be checked by an expert every six months or so if you have high blood pressure.

Check out the stuff on salt on page 4 as salt is one of the major causes of high blood pressure and easy to cut down on. Stop shaking the shaker!

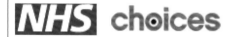 **choices**

Health Checks
It's free and fun, and the right choice for men's tickers.

Activity

Around 100,000 UK men die every year before they reach even the age of 70. That's one man every 4 1/2 minutes. Some men can run a mile in under that time.

Lack of physical activity, together with poor diet, has led to more than 1 in 5 men in England now being seriously overweight. A further 40% are overweight. Diabetes caused by obesity is increasing fast. Diabetes is one of the single most common causes of erectile dysfunction (ED or impotence). Being up for it may be a bigger problem than you think.

Routine maintenance

Men who increase their activity level over a five year period cut their chances of dying early by almost half. Walking instead of using the car helps your health, your bank balance and the environment. Exercise will make you feel better, make you look better and who knows... maybe even make you more attractive (showers permitting!).

Of course, many jobs require lots of exercise. But if yours doesn't, there are simple things you can consider doing to make exercise part of your normal working day. And what better way to start than with the journey to work in the morning?

Travelling to and from work

The journey to work is an ideal chance to help build up the 30 minutes a day of regular physical activity you need. It also has added benefits, as you could save on petrol, fares and commuter stress.

Walking or cycling to work (or to the station if you have a longer journey), instead of driving or using public transport, could make a huge difference. If it takes you 15 minutes each way, you would immediately achieve your recommended daily amount of exercise – and it may even take less time than battling through the traffic.

If your employer doesn't already have schemes in place, ask if they can help to encourage walking and cycling to work.

At work

There are a number of simple things you can do during the work day to stay active – and remember the little things add up!

- Take the stairs instead of the lift; if you work on the top floor, get off a few floors early
- Take opportunities to walk around the office: deliver documents or messages to co-workers in person rather than by email
- Go for a walk at lunch time and during breaks
- Maybe join a sports team for lunchtime or after work.

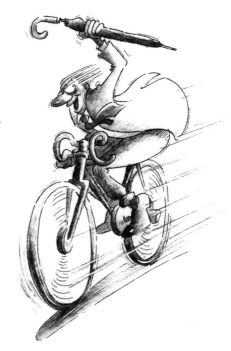

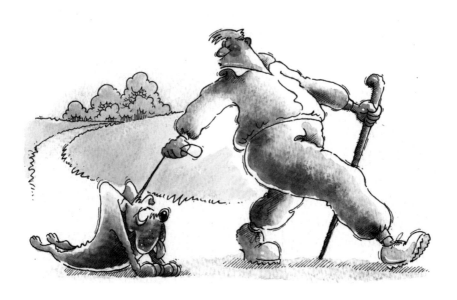

Booze

Lower risk drinking means no more than 3 to 4 units a day for men. If you keep to these amounts you will help prevent damaging your health. (If you're not sure what a unit of alcohol is, check out the table *Just how heavy is your drinking?*)

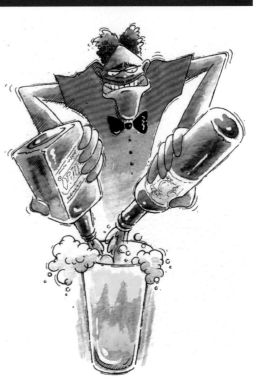

If you regularly drink more than 35 units a week you might already have experienced problems like feeling tired or depressed, putting on weight, memory loss, sleeping badly and having sexual problems. You could also suffer from high blood pressure. Some people are argumentative if they drink a lot, which can affect their relationships with family and friends.

See www.malehealth.co.uk/ drinking

Just how heavy is your drinking?

Large glass of wine (175 millilitres) 15%	3 units	120 to 170 calories
Small glass of wine (125 millilitres) 12%	1½ units	85 to 120 calories
Bottle of wine (750 millilitres) 12%	9 units	510 to 720 calories
Pint of beer 5%	3 units	180 calories
Pint of beer 3.5%	2 units	160 to 170 calories
Single measure of spirits (25 millilitres) 40%	1 unit	60 to 75 calories

---

For more information go to www.drinkaware.co.uk or call 0800 917 8282

Drinking tips

- Walk to the pub to burn off some extra calories on the way
- Drink plenty of water, both during the day and when drinking alcohol
- Try to drink after a meal instead of before – you won't spoil your appetite and you won't feel like drinking so much after your meal
- Try reducing the strength of what you drink. For example, if you normally drink 5% beer, try 3.5% beer instead
- Try to have at least 2 alcohol-free days a week
- A glass of water before your meal may help you both eat and drink less.

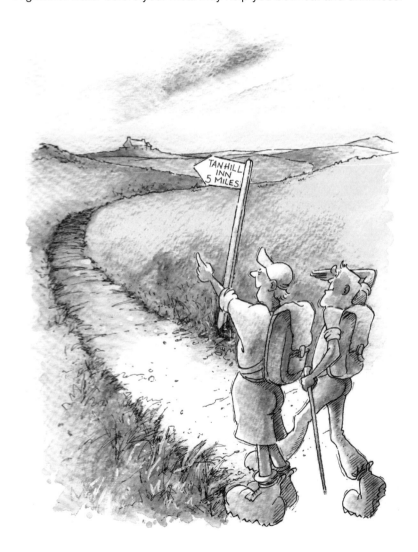

Quitting smoking

Smoking is the single greatest cause of death in the developed world. It has killed more people than both world wars put together – and still kills 114,000 people each year in the UK, commonly through lung cancer and heart disease. One in ten moderate smokers and almost one in five heavy smokers (more than 15 cigarettes a day) will die of lung cancer.

Half of all smokers will die early!

Smokers tend to develop coronary thrombosis (heart attacks) ten years earlier than non-smokers, and account for the vast majority of heart bypass patients. They also take 25% more sick days per year than non-smokers.

On a more positive note, the very moment you stop smoking your health will start to improve. After only 20 minutes of not smoking, your blood pressure and pulse return to normal. In just 48 hours, your body is nicotine-free and carbon monoxide is cleared from your system. And, within 2 to 12 weeks, your circulation improves and you feel noticeably fitter. Best of all, within 5 years your risk of lung cancer will have dropped dramatically, and your risk may be halved by the time you reach your 10th year of being cigarette-free.

Some people try to reduce their cigarette intake gradually. The trouble with this approach is that, as soon as something disturbs your concentration, the numbers tend to creep back up again. It's much better to stop.

Make sure you are ready to give up. Many fail because they jump into the task before they are ready. Have a 'quit plan' and make use of all the sources of help; the NHS offers free help and support for people who want to stop smoking, and there are many other places you can turn to for help.

Ways to help you quit smoking:

- Set a day in advance that you will stop – and tell all your friends, family and workmates so they can support you

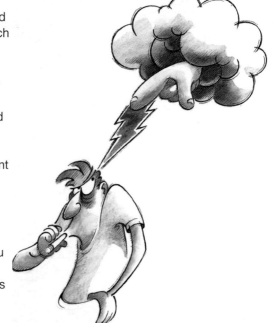

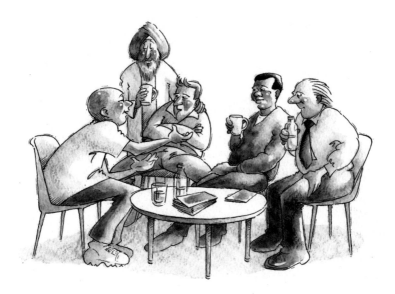

- Do it with a friend or colleague. If someone else gives up with you, you will reinforce each other's willpower; maybe you can get some of your workmates to give up at the same time
- Clear the house (and your car, and desk, and anywhere else you keep them) of all your smoking materials – not just cigarettes, but lighters and matches, rolling papers, ashtrays, etc
- Chew on a carrot – not just good for your health anyway (another of your 5-a-day), but it will also give you something to do with your mouth and hands
- Ask your friends not to smoke around you (or at least pretend they're not enjoying it) – people accept this far more readily than they used to
- Take things one day at a time, and mark your progress on a chart or calendar
- Keep all the money you've saved somewhere safe – and then treat yourself with it
- Make use of any prescription or non-prescription aids available (your pharmacist or GP can advise you on this); or maybe try alternative therapies like hypnotherapy or acupuncture
- Join a 'stop-smoking' support group for professional advice and support from other people

> ### *Did you know?*
> Smokers are at least 50% more likely to have erection problems than non-smokers.

Early warning signs – erectile dysfunction (ED)

There is a close link between:

- Heart disease
- Circulation problems
- Low levels of testosterone
- Diabetes
- Erectile dysfunction.

Getting checked out for all five at the same time might just save your life, let alone your embarrassment.

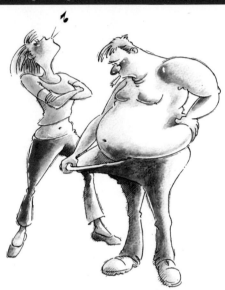

Hard & Fast – hands only CPR

It's in your hands

If an adult has suddenly collapsed, is not breathing normally and is unresponsive, their heart may have stopped beating (cardiac arrest). Doing something, even if untrained, is better than doing nothing.

There are simple actions you can do to help save their life.

- Tell someone to call 999 immediately. If on your own, do this first
- Put the person on their back
- Push hard and fast in the centre of their chest about 100 to 120 times a minute (about the same beat as 'Staying alive') until the ambulance service arrives.

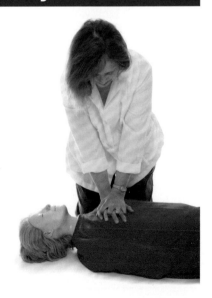

Useful contacts

Fast, free, independent advice from the Men's Health Forum:
www.malehealth.co.uk

NHS - Top 10 healthy heart tips:
http://www.nhs.uk/Livewell/Healthyhearts/Pages/Healthy-heart-tips.aspx

The British Heart Foundation:
http://www.bhf.org.uk/

Drinkaware:
www.drinkaware.co.uk/facts/factsheets/?alcohol-and-men

National Heart Forum:
www.heartforum.org.uk

The Stroke Association:
http://www.stroke.org.uk/

Quit:
www.quit.org.uk

Bandolier:
www.medicine.ox.ac.uk/bandolier (Coronary Heart Disease)

Pulmonary Hypertension Association UK:
www.phassociation.uk.com

Net Doctor:
www.netdoctor.co.uk/diseases/facts/impotence.htm

London Urology Associates:
www.lua.co.uk/erectile-dysfunction/what-causes-impotence

Physical Activity:
www.patient.co.uk/health/Physical-Activity-For-Health.htm

NHS Choices:
www.nhs.uk/

Malehealth
the first choice for men's health info

Malehealth, the MHF's health information website for men, has had over three million visitors in the last two years. Why? Because it's fast, it's free and it's independent. Penises to prostates, alcohol to ageing, lungs to livers, hearts to hormones – whatever your question on male health, you'll find the answer at

www.malehealth.co.uk.

ISBN 978 0 85761 034 8

9 780857 610348

Publication of Men's Health Forum

Haynes Publishing, Sparkford, Yeovil,
Somerset BA22 7JJ England

32-36 Loman Street,
London SE1 0EH

www.haynes.co.uk   www.menshealthforum.co.uk